INTRODUCTION

What do you do when you have been obese for all of your life? You've been teased, ridiculed, and tormented for your big size, and you feel like there is nothing you can do about it. You have tried on numerous occasions to lose some of the weight; you've experimented with countless numbers of diets and even enrolled in a few exercise programs at the gym but alas, nothing has worked in the long run because you are still obese. You feel despondent now because you feel like nothing can help your plight. You believe that it is your fault; you believe that your gluttony has caused your corpulence, and you believe that you will be fat forever. What if I told you that maybe it isn't your fault at all? What if I told you that maybe a hormonal imbalance has been the cause of your obesity and that you may be Leptin-resistant?

This hormone that was discovered in 1994 has revolutionized the way many scientists and experts alike look at the condition of obesity. Instead of looking at this disease through censuring lens, scientists are finally looking at obesity in an unbiased manner and realizing that Leptin, often dubbed as the satiety hormone, may contribute to this debilitating disease similar to the way insulin contributes to diabetes.

Read on if you are finally ready to let go of all your self-pity and self-loathing; if you are ready to learn about obesity and take effective steps to lose the weight forever, then this is the book for you.

First things first: What is Leptin?

To fully understand what Leptin is and its function in the body, we have to go way back in the day. We have to go back to the time when the human race knew nothing about farming. We have to go back to the days when we were hunters and gatherers. Back then, when the summer was in, many fruits were in season and many edible animals were running about—we would have a feast! We would eat a lot of food in preparation for the winter because that season brought with it nothing but starvation. During the winter, the fruit trees stopped producing their wonderful fruit and most animals hibernated, so there wasn't much food to go around. Yet, we had to be careful during our summer feasts to not overeat because if we did, we would get fat, and being obese was just as bad in those times as starving because both conditions made it more difficult to survive in the natural environment. Both conditions, obesity and starvation, were two extremes to be avoided, and the hormone Leptin was produced in our bodies to ensure that the delicate balance between the two was maintained. It caused us to get hungrier and eat when our fat stores were being used up (i.e. when we were starting to starve), but it also forced us to stop eating when our fat stores were getting too large (i.e. when we were putting on too much weight) and bordering on the line of obesity.

Therefore, Leptin tells the hypothalamus of our brains when we have enough energy stored in our bodies. When we have enough energy stored, that means that we do not need to eat extra food to build up those energy stores, it means that we can burn calories at a normal rate, and it also means that we can engage in energy-expensive processes like pregnancy and puberty.

Energy is stored in our bodies in the form of fat, so it makes sense that the fat cells are the ones that produce Leptin. As you can imagine, each of us has our own specific energy thresholds because everyone's body is different and everyone has their own specific needs.

Therefore, when we are at a normal weight, our fat cells will be producing a certain quantity of Leptin, and our brains (specifically our hypothalamuses) will register that amount as the threshold—the normal and healthy amount to be produced. When we start to lose weight, however, it means that we will have less fat cells in our bodies and hence less producers of Leptin. With less Leptin being produced, that means that we will be below our threshold and the brain will set mechanisms in place to have us eating more food to replenish those fat stores and also have us using up less energy so that less fat will be burned. This will help to prevent starvation.

In the same way, if we are eating too much food, then the amount of Leptin in our bodies will be above the threshold. To prevent obesity, our brains will decrease our appetite and make us engage in more energy-expensive activities so that we can lose the extra fat and be back to the normal balance again.

These concepts can more easily be understood by consulting the diagrams on the following pages.

When We Lose Weight and Go Below the Optimum Weight/Threshold

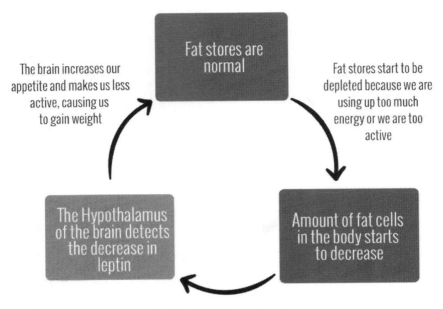

When we gain weight and go above our optimum weight

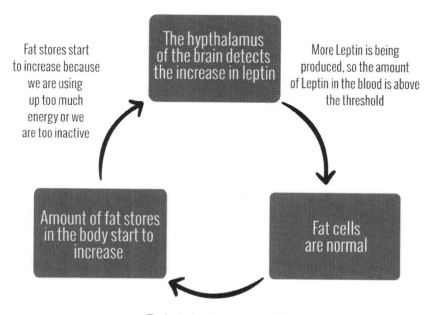

In people who are Leptin-resistant, something else happens: instead of detecting the quantities of Leptin in their blood, their hypothalamuses are "blind" to it and do not make the necessary changes to reduce the appetite and increase bodily activity. This will be explained further in the next section.

WHAT IS LEPTIN RESISTANCE AND HOW IT WORKS

Before we go into an in-depth explanation of what Leptin resistance really is, let us summarize what we have learned so far:

- Leptin is the hormone that controls energy expenditure in humans. It tells the hypothalamus of the brain when we have enough energy stored, and this causes the brain to decrease our appetite until we are back to normal. It also tells the hypothalamus of the brain when we have too little energy, and our brains will increase our appetite and make us eat more so that we can replenish our energy stores.
- Leptin is produced by the fat cells of our bodies. The more we gain weight, the more fat cells we have, and therefore the more Leptin we produce. The more we lose weight, the less fat cells we have, and the less Leptin we produce.
- In Leptin-resistant people, the hypothalamus of their brains are "blind" to the quantity of Leptin in the blood, so Leptin is unable to produce its normal effects on the hypothalamus, which is therefore unable to make changes to our appetite and/or activity to cause us to lose the excess weight.

I'm sure you're wondering exactly what I mean when I say the brain is blind, and it is time I tell you. Our bodies are filled with receptors that help us to detect certain changes and substances in our

Leptin Resistance

internal and external environment. There is a receptor for blood pressure, a receptor for blood glucose levels, and a receptor for blood Leptin levels. During Leptin resistance, something blocks these blood Leptin receptors and makes them less receptive to the stimulus of Leptin. Therefore, the Leptin receptors erroneously report back to the brain a lesser amount of Leptin than what is actually present in the blood.

The Leptin receptors can be so defective that the amount of Leptin that they report back to the brain is similar to the amount that would be reported if the body were in starvation mode. This causes the brain to put mechanisms in place to prevent starvation because, as you already know, starvation can be one of the most dangerous things to befall the human body. This is exactly what happens in people who are obese. They have excessive amounts of fat cells in their bodies, and these fat cells are producing excessive amounts of Leptin, but the receptors are not detecting the correct quantities of Leptin floating around in the blood and are reporting an erroneous figure back to the brain. Hence, the bodies of Leptin-resistant obese people are reporting that they are obese, but the brain believes that it is starving.

When the brain receives these low Leptin reports from the Leptin receptors, it frantically tries to save the person by increasing the appetite so that more fats can be stored, and it also makes the person less active so that less energy can be expended. This action of the brain is the exact reason why obese people have such huge appetites and why they are usually so inactive and sleepy too. It is their brains' desperate attempts to save themselves from starvation and ultimately death.

Obese people, therefore, find it very hard to override the commands of their brains by going on diets or exercising and, in fact, this can actually make the situation worse. Remember that the brain is getting an erroneously low figure for the amount of Leptin floating around in the blood. When an obese person starts to exercise or go on a diet, they are actually causing more fat cells to be depleted, so an even lesser amount of Leptin is being reported back to the brain! The brain, therefore, launches a panic attack and puts all of its energy into regaining that lost energy, i.e. fat. Therefore, the obese person's appetite will double, maybe even triple, as the brain tries to save the person from what it believes to be the last lap of starvation before death occurs. The person will also feel more tired and sleepy, and instead of wanting to exercise, they will feel like just lying down and sleeping—this is the brain's attempt to get the body to move less so that less energy will be expended.

"But what could cause the Leptin receptors to be so unresponsive in the first place?" you might ask; after all, if they weren't making erroneous reports to the brain, no one would have this problem. Read on to the next section where we shall explore the reason behind such unresponsive Leptin receptors.

Causes of Leptin Resistance

To fully understand what causes Leptin resistance, it makes sense to call to memory a story you may have heard some time ago when you were a child—the story of the boy who cried wolf. The first time he cried wolf, he got the attention of all the villagers, but the more he continued to do this, the less attention he got from the villagers, until one day all the villagers became totally unresponsive to his calls because they got used to his silly pranks.

It is a similar case with Leptin resistance. The Leptin receptors are so used to being bombarded by so many Leptin molecules that they become overwhelmed and shut down to protect themselves. It is like the body is crying, "Leptin, Leptin, Leptin!" but the receptors have gotten so used to detecting that high amount of Leptin in the blood that they become desensitized and do not transmit the signal to the brain. The signal does not get to the brain to tell it to stop eating so much, so the problem of Leptin resistance develops. Therefore, an obese and Leptin-resistant person has to eat more and more food to feel satiated, and the more food he or she eats, the more fats get stored and the more Leptin gets produced, and this greater quantity of Leptin floating around in the blood will cause even more of the Leptin receptors to lose their sensitivity. As you can imagine, this forms a vicious cycle of an increased appetite and constant hunger, increased weight gain due to more fat storage, and a decreased sensitivity to the hormone Leptin.

Diets

There are other factors that can affect the Leptin receptors in the body. Diets that are high in fats and simple carbohydrates can greatly affect the Leptin receptors and hinder them from doing their jobs. The Western diet is filled with foods that have been sweetened by simple sugars (usually sucrose and fructose) and unhealthy fats. You would be surprised to realize that even foods that have been marketed as being healthy and good for you have been stuffed with large amounts of saturated fats, high fructose corn syrup, and other dangerous sweeteners that are high in energy but low in everything else.

One molecule of sucrose is made up of one molecule of glucose and one molecule of fructose. Both sugars have the same chemical formula, but fructose is metabolized in the body in a completely different way than glucose. When glucose is ingested, it can be utilized by any cell in the body directly for energy. It is used to make other sugars that are needed in your genetic material, and it can also be used to make protein-sugar complexes that constitute your lubricating fluids and connective tissues. When there are excess amounts of glucose in the body, some of it is converted to glycogen, and when the glycogen stores have been filled, the rest of the glucose is converted to fats.

When fructose is ingested, it takes a completely different route. It is metabolized only by the cells of the liver and converted to triglycerides, free radicals, and uric acid. Having high levels of free radicals and uric acid in the blood can have dangerous repercussions on various systems of the body, but when there is a high concentration of fructose molecules, they can actually block the Leptin receptors directly, thereby preventing the message of satiety from being carried to the brain. This contributes to even more Leptin resistance. The triglycerides that are produced when the fructose is broken down can also interfere with the Leptin receptors, and even if they do not do that, when they are stored, they still become a part of the body's fat cells and help to produce even more Leptin which further desensitizes the Leptin receptors.

In summary, large amounts of sugars like sucrose raise the quantity of glucose which floats around in the blood; this may lead to insulin resistance, which is another related complication that will be discussed further down in the book. The excess glucose that is in the blood may also be converted to bodily fats (also called triglycerides) which will help to produce even more Leptin and make the body more Leptin-resistant than it already is. Fructose molecules block the Leptin receptors directly, and when they break down, they form triglycerides which also interfere with the Leptin receptors and help to make up fat cells which will produce even more excess Leptin, further contributing to the problem of Leptin resistance.

High fat diets, especially those high in saturated fats, also pose this same risk of causing Leptin resistance because they add so much extra triglycerides to the body.

Hormones

The hormone insulin is also cited as a culprit in the Leptin resistance saga, but this is still linked to a high sugar intake. Whenever we ingest large quantities of sugars, our blood insulin levels rise as the hormone removes excess sugars from the blood. It aids body cells by helping them to absorb glucose from the blood and also signals the liver to take up some of the glucose and store it as glycogen. When the glycogen stores have been filled, insulin signals the fat cells to take up the glucose and store it as triglycerides; this thereby adds more fats to the body.

Insulin and Leptin resistance are related because the high sugar levels that cause the Leptin receptors to be unresponsive also cause the insulin receptors to be unresponsive. Therefore, a large quantity of glucose is left in the blood, and a large quantity of insulin is being produced by the body as well because the glucose is not being absorbed. High levels of insulin prevent us from burning body fat and, in fact, induce even more fat storage. This extra fat produces even more Leptin hormone which further aggravates the Leptin resistance and leads to further overeating, raising blood glucose levels even more. Insulin may also help to block the Leptin receptors and render them unresponsive to relaying the message of satiety in the brain. A vicious cycle of overeating and weight gain then ensues.

Stress

The hormone cortisol is the hormone released during times of stress. In the short term, it causes blood glucose levels to rise and causes fat to be converted to energy, leading to a decrease in the amount of fat cells. This means that Leptin levels will decrease during times of stress in the short term. People usually increase their food intake in relation to stress when the stress factor is prolonged; therefore, in the long term, stress causes us to gain more fat and, therefore, produce more Leptin. If the stress continues to rise and is not dealt with, it will continue to raise the blood Leptin levels and Leptin resistance will follow suit shortly after.

Signs of Leptin resistance

The first and most obvious sign of Leptin resistance would definitely be being overweight. Scientists agree that if someone is obese, then there is almost a 100% chance that they are Leptin-resistant. Constant fatigue is also another common symptom in people who are Leptin-resistant.

Having a big appetite and carbohydrate cravings, especially at night, is also another common sign that someone is Leptin-resistant. This huge appetite usually leads to overeating, so if you see someone who is always over-eating, then it is very much likely that they are Leptin-resistant.

Having a high level of stress, being irritable, or having mood swings may also be a sign that someone is Leptin-resistant. Having high blood sugar, coupled with high triglycerides and high cholesterol, may also mean that you are Leptin-resistant.

Thyroid problems, liver problems, and reproductive problems are also very common in people who are Leptin-resistant.

Treating Leptin Resistance Naturally

Habits and Actions to adopt and avoid:

Proper Stress Management

You have seen the effect that unhealthy and prolonged stress has on the hormonal balance in the body. It leads to a myriad of complications which all work in unison to make the Leptin resistance worse. So, to reduce your Leptin resistance and eventually eliminate it, you need to take steps to reduce or remove the stress factors in your life. A few minutes each day of meditation can go a long way in easing anxiety or any other stress factors that may be getting you down. Simply close your eyes and repeat a positive mantra like "I love myself" or "I am at peace" and let any distracting thought float away with each breath you exhale. Taking five minute breaks to breathe in deeply can also help you relax. Deep breathing helps to negate the effects of stress by lowering your blood pressure and slowing your heart rate. Talking with close friends and family can also help to remove some stress and anxiety. Give them a shout, find out about their days; just being in the company of someone you care about can go a long way in reducing your stress and anxiety and thereby reducing your Leptin resistance.

Exercise the right way

Have you ever wondered why your appetite decreases over time with moderate physical activity? Yeah, that right! Your appetite decreases because exercise mitigates the effect that cortisol has on your body and reduces your Leptin resistance.

Start slowly when you decide to add exercise to your regular routine because the body would consider strenuous exercise to be a form of stress on the body, and this would only make your Leptin resistance worse. Avoid cardio when you just start exercising; instead, opt for resistance (weight) training. Remember if you are Leptin-resistant, your brain is in starvation mode, so it will refuse to burn its "low" energy stores to feed your muscles—even if you need it. So, doing cardio which demands a lot of energy would not have any positive effects on your body when you have just started. Resistance training will cause your body to produce growth hormones, which would restart your metabolism and cause your body to start burning energy to supply your muscles. After you have started losing weight and your cravings have started to decrease, then you can add cardio to your exercise routine because that would mean that your metabolism is up and running and your body is willing to burn fat. You should also consider working out in the mid-afternoon or evening to support hormone levels.

Get adequate amounts of sleep

Sleep is critical for general health and metabolism but it is extremely important for the reversal of Leptin resistance and here is why: sleep helps you lose weight, sleep improves your performance at everything you do, and sleep helps to restore and rejuvenate your tissues. Consistently getting less than six hours of sleep nightly makes it harder for you to lose weight. This is because during sleep, your body secretes hormones that regulate your blood sugar levels and your appetite. Insufficient sleep decreases the hormone Leptin and increases cortisol; this thereby increases the amount of sugar circulating in the blood. Constantly having a high concentration of sugar in your blood will inevitably lead to weight gain because insulin will cause the excesses to be converted to fat. It may eventually lead to poor blood sugar control and even diabetes.

Getting adequate amounts of sleep will also improve your performance in everything you do. When we are awake, a substance known as adenosine (a by-product of neuronal activity) is produced in our bodies and builds up until we sleep. It leads to us feeling drowsy, and everyone knows that you are less efficient when you are drowsy than when you are fully rested. Therefore, with proper rest you will be better able to complete your weight training and eventually your cardio; this will help you lose the weight and keep it off. You will also do better at every other activity in your life, and this will boost your confidence and reduce your stress levels as well.

Finally, sleep helps to restore your tissues and rejuvenate them too. While most physiological activities are decreased during sleep, the release of growth hormone into the blood stream isn't. Growth hormone helps to repair tissues, especially muscles, from the wear and tear of everyday life. Stronger muscles mean that you will be better able to undertake more physical activity which will help to get your metabolism back up and running again. Restoring your normal metabolic rate is one of the most important things that you can do to reduce your Leptin resistance, so ensure that you get adequate sleep at night.

Eat every three to four hours

You should try to space out your meals so that they are at least three to four hours apart. This includes drinks that have calories, but tea without sugar or cream, coffee, water, and herbal teas are fine. You should also ensure that you have three meals a day, and there should be no snacking in between meals. This will help to get your hormones balanced again. When you constantly eat throughout the day, your liver doesn't get a chance to rest so that your hormonal levels can go back to normal again, so avoid snacking at all costs. You can safely lower your Leptin levels by engaging in intermittent fasting if you like.

Avoid very low calorie diets

By now you should know that very low calorie diets should be avoided if your aim is to reduce your Leptin resistance. Low calorie diets would be those that restrict you to one thousand calories or less daily. This would only put stress on the body, raise your cortisol levels, and cause you to gain even more weight; your body would go into overdrive as it tries to protect you from "starvation." Low calorie diets would cause hormonal surges in your body, and that would only lead to uncontrollable hunger, so ensure that you stay away from those very low calorie diets.

Avoid MSG (monosodium glutamate) and aspartame

Monosodium glutamate and aspartame will lead you down a path of obesity, metabolic syndrome, and diabetes, and it will make your appetite spiral out of control. Monosodium glutamate and aspartame are added to 80% of all flavored foods. They excite the area of your brain that is responsible for fat metabolism and fat storage, and experiments have even proven that they can scar the hypothalamus and lead to what is known as hypothalamic obesity. By scarring your hypothalamus, monosodium glutamate and aspartame disrupt your fat metabolism and cause you to gain weight. This extra fat thereby produces more Leptin which eventually leads to Leptin resistance, and with a defective hypothalamus and excess Leptin at play, your weight will inevitably spiral out of control. Monosodium glutamate and aspartame are also known to raise blood insulin levels. This also leads to insulin resistance, diabetes, and a myriad of problems after that.

Take in more omega-3 fatty acids and reduce your omega-6 fatty acids

Leptin resistance, insulin resistance, and other complications resulting from hormonal imbalances are simply inflammations in the body. You can reduce these inflammations by increasing the amounts of omega-3 fatty acids that you consume and by reducing the amounts of omega-6 fatty acids that you consume. Omega-3 fatty acids help to support healthy Leptin levels by helping to repair Leptin receptors that have been desensitized. Omega-6 fatty acids do the opposite and help to make the Leptin receptors even more desensitized. Therefore, eat foods that are high in omega-3 fatty acids. These foods include kale, summer squash, flax seeds, chia seeds, trout, mackerel, sardines, anchovies, salmon, walnuts, and grass-fed meats. Foods to avoid are vegetable oils, conventional meats, and grains because they contain a substantial amount of omega-6 fatty acids.

Eat more proteins

It is recommended that you eat proteins at every meal, especially at breakfast. It is very effective at improving Leptin sensitivity, and it also takes a longer time to digest. Therefore, it will keep you feeling full for a long period of time. Proteins also slow down the release of glucose into the blood stream, so they will lessen the great hormonal surges that occur when we eat and help to control and reduce the onset of diabetes. Another thing about protein is that it increases your metabolism by as much as 30% for half a day or less. This is the calorie-burning equivalent of a two- or three-mile run. Restarting your metabolism and getting it back to normal is one of the most important things for you to achieve if you want to regain Leptin sensitivity. Proteins can really help you to achieve your goal and get you back into perfect health.

Cut back on those high carbohydrate foods, refined foods, and sugary foods

You may think that the easiest way to rectify your Leptin resistance would be to cut carbohydrates out of your diet completely, but that sort of thinking is wrong! Cutting carbohydrates out of your body would only make you less healthy; your muscles would weaken, your digestive system would be compromised, growth hormone would not be released properly, your heart would become stressed, your electrolytes would become unregulated, your fat would not burn efficiently, and your thyroid gland would shut down! Avoiding carbohydrates completely would not be the answer at all because carbohydrates themselves are not bad. It is just the quantities and types of carbohydrates that we consume that cause problems.

Most overweight and obese people eat double or even triple the amounts of carbohydrates that their bodies need. As such, their bodies store the excess carbohydrates as fats and these ever-increasing fat stores produce more Leptin and lead to Leptin resistance. To accurately determine how many carbohydrates you should be ingesting, you should look at the food on your plate and use the 50/50 technique. You should have a palm-sized portion of proteins (six to eight ounce portion for men or a four to six ounce portion for women), and you should also see a palm-sized portion for carbohydrates. That is the 50/50 technique. You should also have lots of fiber-rich vegetables and moderate amounts of fruits.

You should endeavor to eat large quantities of foods high in fiber at every meal. That includes vegetables and some fruits. Fiber-rich foods will help to fill up your tummy quickly and make you less likely to overeat. You will feel fuller, and what's more, those high fiber foods usually do not have too many calories either. This will help to stabilize your hormones, and, over time, it will help to reduce your Leptin and insulin sensitivity and bring you back to normal health.

You should cut back on refined foods and sugary foods because more than likely they contain fructose and other sweeteners that will only damage your hormonal balance even more. In fact, you should avoid fructose and those other sweeteners like the plague! You already know the effect that high fructose ingestion has on the body and the reasons why it damages your Leptin sensitivity. Fruits are also a source of fructose, but fruits often contain antioxidants, fiber, and other helpful substances that will slow down the release of fructose into the blood and also help to reverse any damages that it may cause. Fruits usually do not contain such large concentrations of fructose anyway, so eating some fruit should not be a major concern; just do not overdo it. Twenty-five grams or one piece of fruit of fruit per day would be fine. You should also be concerned about the fructose content in fruit juices and dried fruits, which are often modified to raise their sugar content and make them more palatable.

Take Supplements

There are many supplements out there that will help to reduce your Leptin resistance; you just have to choose the right one. Fucoxanthin is a carotenoid that has been used for ages to reduce inflammation, and it has shown positive results in reducing Leptin resistance too. It can be found in brown seaweed, but you can also take fucoxanthin supplements and reap the same benefits.

Zinc has also proven useful in the fight against Leptin resistance. It has been proven to bolster the performance of Leptin and help it work at optimal levels in the body. Some major sources of zinc include lamb, pork, beef, fish, chicken, and yeast. Another supplement to consider is one that heals your intestines and therefore helps to control your body weight and your appetite. It has been used to treat the intestines because of its healing properties. I am talking about probiotics. Probiotics are the beneficial bacteria that live inside our digestive tract. They can also be found in many food sources. Doctors have realized that when the ratio of probiotics falls below 85% along the intestinal tract, many health issues arise, including Leptin resistance. Probiotics have been shown to reduce Leptin concentrations in the body and have been used to help gut disorders such as colitis. So, eat bone broths and take probiotics to heal your intestinal walls. Some good sources of probiotics include sauerkraut, miso, kimchi, tempeh, kombucha, kefir, pickled/fermented vegetables, sourdough bread, natto, soft cheeses, and yogurt. You can also take probiotic supplements. Foods that contain inulin, including bananas, sun-chokes, artichokes, leeks, onions, and garlic, feed the good gut bacteria and promote their replication and are therefore just as effective as taking probiotic supplements.

Extracts of the irvingia gabonensis plant have also been making headway in helping obese people lose and keep off weight, even without other lifestyle altercations. It has also shown promising results in helping people regain Leptin sensitivity and reverse the effects of cellular inflammation. It has had a positive impact on other hormonal systems, including that of adiponectin and insulin.

This plant extract was used in many experiments to inhibit the action of the digestive enzyme that is used to break down complex carbohydrates into simple sugars. This thereby slows down the rate at which glucose enters the bloodstream and hence prevents the rapid hormonal surges that would have occurred without the irvingia gabonensis. It also helps to inhibit the hormone that facilitates the conversion of blood glucose into triglycerides or bodily fat. This reduces the amount of glucose in the blood that is converted to fats, and you can see how this benefits Leptin resistance. If you could get some of the fruit of the irvingia gabonensis plant or extracts of it, it would go a long way in reducing your Leptin resistance and helping to get you healthy again.

Avoid lectins

Cereal grains such as rye, barley, and wheat contain a substance known as wheat germ agglutinin, or WGA, which is a type of lectin. Lectins are substances that plants produce to protect themselves from diseases and insects. This substance actually binds to the Leptin receptors directly and so prevents the Leptin hormone from binding to them and stimulating them. This obviously contributes to Leptin resistance. Therefore, avoid cereal grains, legumes, soy, and peanuts as much as possible, until you regain your Leptin sensitivity, because they contain large quantities of lectin.

Meal Ideas

After reading so many of the do's and don'ts for reducing Leptin resistance, you may feel overwhelmed and may think that you may never be able to plan the right meals that will adhere to the rules given above. Some of you may think that the meals you will have to prepare will be boring and bland, but you are wrong! You can still make marvelous meals that are healthy and delicious. Try out the following recipes and make adjustments to them as you like; reversing your Leptin resistance will be as easy as one, two, three with these ambrosial meals.

Breakfast

Paleo Pancakes with Pureed Strawberries

"This Paleo-friendly, flourless pancake recipe is topped with pureed strawberries."

Prep Time: 10 Minutes
Cook Time: 20 Minutes
Ready In: 30 Minutes
Servings: 10

INGREDIENTS:
2 eggs
1 ½ cups almond flour
½ teaspoon ground cinnamon
½ teaspoon vanilla extract

¼ teaspoon baking powder
½ cup applesauce
¼ cup coconut milk, or more as needed
1 teaspoon olive oil, for frying

Topping
1 cup strawberries

DIRECTIONS:

1. Mix together the eggs, almond flour, cinnamon, vanilla extract, baking powder, applesauce, and coconut milk in a bowl.
2. Lightly oil a griddle and put it over medium-high heat.
3. Drop large spoonsful of the batter onto the griddle and cook until the pancake edges become dry and bubbles form.
4. Flip the pancake and allow the other side to cook until it is browned
5. Repeat the procedure with the remaining batter.
6. Puree the strawberries until they become smooth in a food processor.
7. Top the pancakes with the pureed strawberries.

NUTRITIONAL INFORMATION:

Servings Per Recipe: 10
Calories: 112
Amount Per Serving
Total Fat: 5.9g
Cholesterol: 42mg
Sodium: 29mg
Total Carbs: 8.4g
Dietary Fiber: 0.7g
Protein: 8.2g

Bacon Pancakes (Paleo)

"Start your day off right by making your pancakes with a bacon-twist because you know what they say: 'everything's better with bacon!'"

Prep Time: 15 Minutes
Cook Time: 20 Minutes
Ready In: 40 Minutes
Servings: 2

INGREDIENTS:
3 slices bacon
1 banana, chopped
2 eggs
1 teaspoon vanilla extract
1 pinch baking soda
2 tablespoons coconut flour
1 pinch salt
1 pinch baking powder

DIRECTIONS:
1. Place the slices of bacon in a large skillet and cook them over medium-high heat for about 10 minutes whilst turning them occasionally until they are evenly browned.
2. Drain the bacon slices on paper towels and then pour the drippings from the bacon into a glass bowl.
3. Crumble the bacon
4. Beat the banana and eggs in a bowl with an electric mixer until the mixture becomes smooth and foamy.
5. Beat 1 1/2 tablespoons of the bacon drippings and also the crumbled bacon pieces with the vanilla extract, and then stir it into the egg mixture.

6. Whisk baking soda, coconut flour, salt, and baking powder into the egg mixture until the batter is just combined.

7. Allow the batter to stand for 2 minutes.

8. Lightly grease a griddle with the bacon drippings and heat it over medium-high heat.

9. Drop large spoonsful of the batter on to the griddle and cook them until the edges become dry and bubbles start to form in them; this will take 3-4 minutes.

10. Flip the pancakes and cook the other sides for 2-3 minutes or until they are browned.

11. Repeat the procedure with the rest of the batter.

NUTRITIONAL INFORMATION:
Servings Per Recipe: 2
Calories: 264
Amount Per Serving
Total Fat: 12.3g
Cholesterol: 226mg
Sodium: 766mg
Total Carbs: 24.5g
Dietary Fiber: 7.5g
Protein: 13.9g

Paleo Oatmeal (Not Really Oatmeal at All)

"This Paleo-friendly, hearty, hot 'oatmeal' is filled with walnuts, pecans, raisins, and apples."

Prep Time: 10 Minutes
Cook Time: 10 Minutes
Ready In: 20 Minutes
Servings: 2

INGREDIENTS:
1/2 teaspoon pumpkin pie spice
1/2 teaspoon ground cinnamon
1 teaspoon coconut oil
1/2 cup raisins
1 apple, diced
1 splash vanilla extract
1 tablespoon almond butter
1/4 cup almond milk
3 eggs
1 banana
1/4 cup ground pecans, or to taste
1/4 cup ground walnuts, or to taste
1 tablespoon maple syrup, or more to taste

DIRECTIONS:
1. Stir the pumpkin pie spice, cinnamon, coconut oil, raisins, and diced apple together over medium heat in a saucepan.
2. Bring the mixture to a simmer and cook it for about 5 minutes to blend flavors.
3. Blend the vanilla extract, almond butter, almond milk, eggs and the banana together in a food processor.

4. Add the pecans and walnuts to banana mixture and blend them together.

5. Stir the banana mixture and the maple syrup into the apple mixture; bring it to a simmer and cook it for 5-10 minutes or until the mixture becomes thick.

NUTRITIONAL INFORMATION:
Servings Per Recipe: 2
Calories: 615
Amount Per Serving
Total Fat: 35.9g
Cholesterol: 317mg
Sodium: 168mg
Total Carbs: 66.8g
Dietary Fiber: 7.8g
Protein: 16.4g

Paleo Greek 'Rice'

"A delicious Paleo cauliflower 'rice' that is steamed with bell peppers, onions, and tomatoes and then topped with a lemony dressing and mint."

Prep Time: 15 Minutes
Cook Time: 15 Minutes
Ready In: 1 Hour
Servings: 6

INGREDIENTS:
1/4 cup fresh lemon juice
1/2 yellow onion, diced small
1 head cauliflower, cut into large florets
1/2 cup grape tomatoes, halved
1/2 red bell pepper, diced small
3 tablespoons chopped fresh mint
1/4 cup extra virgin olive oil
Ground black pepper, to taste
Salt, to taste

DIRECTIONS:
1. Stir the lemon juice and onion together in a bowl and allow the mixture to rest for half an hour or until the onion flavor mellows.
2. Drain the onion but save the lemon juice.
3. Shred the cauliflower in a food processor until it is the size of small rice grains.
4. Put the cauliflower over medium heat in a skillet.
5. Cover the skillet and cook the cauliflower whilst stirring occasionally for 8-10 minutes or until the cauliflower is fully steamed.
6. Remove the lid from the skillet and stir in the grape tomatoes and the red bell pepper.

7. Cook the mixture whilst stirring occasionally for about 3 minutes or until it is fully heated through.

8. Add the mint and the onion to the cauliflower mixture; stir and cook for about 3 minutes or until the mixture is fully heated through.

9. Whisk 3 tablespoons reserved lemon juice, the olive oil, the black pepper and the salt together in a bowl.

10. Pour the lemon juice mixture over cauliflower mixture and toss it to coat it.

11. Finally, season the Greek rice with black pepper and salt to taste.

NUTRITIONAL INFORMATION:
Servings Per Recipe: 6
Calories: 120
Amount Per Serving
Total Fat: 9.5g
Cholesterol: 0mg
Sodium: 95mg
Total Carbs: 8g
Dietary Fiber: 2.9g
Protein: 2.3g

Lunch

Paleo Salmon Burgers

"Salmon burgers made with parsley and gluten-free bread crumbs can fit into any Paleo or gluten-free diet."

Prep Time: 10 Minutes
Cook Time: 10 Minutes
Ready In: 20 Minutes
Servings: 8

INGREDIENTS:
1/4 teaspoon garlic salt
2 teaspoons lemon juice
1 tablespoon fresh parsley, chopped
3 tablespoons mayonnaise
2 eggs, beaten
1/2 cup onions, chopped
1 cup gluten-free bread crumbs
1 can (14 ounce) salmon, drained and flaked
1 tablespoon olive oil, or more as needed

DIRECTIONS:
1. Mix the garlic salt, lemon juice, parsley, mayonnaise, eggs, onions, bread crumbs, and salmon together in a bowl.
2. Form the mixture into patties.
3. Heat the olive oil over medium heat in a skillet or a grill-pan.
4. Cook the patties for about 5 minutes per side or until they are browned.

NUTRITIONAL INFORMATION:
Servings Per Recipe: 2

Ella Marie

Calories: 556
Amount Per Serving
Total Fat: 53.6g
Cholesterol: 0mg
Sodium: 9mg
Total Carbs: 17.6g
Dietary Fiber: 7.2g
Protein: 11.2g

Paleo Banana Bread

"This gluten-free, Paleo-friendly banana bread is moist and dense."

Prep Time: 15 Minutes
Cook Time: 45 Minutes
Ready In: 1 Hour
Servings: 12

INGREDIENTS:
1 serving cooking spray
1 teaspoon baking soda
1 tablespoon ground cinnamon
2 cups almond flour
2 eggs
1/2 cup water
1 teaspoon almond extract
1/4 cup agave syrup
2 bananas, ripe and mashed
1/2 teaspoon vanilla bean paste, optional

DIRECTIONS:
1. Preheat the oven to a temperature of 350°F (175°C).
2. Spray the loaf pan with some cooking spray.
3. Mix together the baking soda, ground cinnamon, and almond flour in a bowl.
4. Beat the eggs in a bowl
5. Mix in the vanilla bean paste, mashed bananas, agave syrup, almond extract, and water.
6. Mix the banana mixture into the almond flour mixture until no dry areas remain.
7. Pour the batter into the loaf pan that you prepared before.

8. Bake the banana bread in the preheated oven for about 45 minutes or until the bread is brown and crisp around the edges.

NUTRITIONAL INFORMATION:
Servings Per Recipe: 12
Calories: 127
Amount Per Serving
Total Fat: 4.3g
Cholesterol: 31mg
Sodium: 117mg
Total Carbs: 15.8g
Dietary Fiber: 1.1g
Protein: 8.6g

Italian Paleo Chicken Meat Loaf

"This Italian-inspired chicken meatloaf makes a tasty yet simple lunch, and it is Paleo-friendly too."

Prep Time: 15 Minutes
Cook Time: 2 Hours
Ready In: 2 Hours 35 Minutes
Servings: 8

INGREDIENTS:
1 teaspoon ground black pepper
1 tablespoon Italian seasoning
2 garlic cloves
1/4 large onion
1 celery stalk
6 carrots
7 chicken tenderloins
4 eggs
1 can (8 ounce) tomato sauce, no-salt-added and divided

DIRECTIONS:
1. Preheat the oven to a temperature of 350°F (175°C).
2. Grease a 9x5-inch loaf pan.
3. Put the black pepper, Italian seasoning, garlic, onion, celery, and carrots in a food processor and mince them.
4. Take the vegetable mixture out of the food processor and put it in a large bowl.
5. Place the chicken tenderloins in the food processor and process them until they are grounded.
6. Use a fork to mix the eggs into the vegetable mixture until they are fully incorporated.

7. Then add half the tomato sauce into the mixture and mix again.

8. Fold the chicken into the vegetable-tomato sauce mixture and pour it into the prepared loaf pan.

9. Bake the batter in the preheated oven for one and a half hours.

10. Spread the rest of the tomato sauce over the meatloaf.

11. Bake the meat loaf for about half an hour more or until the meatloaf is cooked through. An instant-read thermometer inserted into the center of the meatloaf should read at least 165°F (74°C).

12. Let the meatloaf cool in the loaf pan for 20 minutes before you attempt to slice it.

NUTRITIONAL INFORMATION:
Servings Per Recipe: 8
Calories: 123
Amount Per Serving
Total Fat: 3.3g
Cholesterol: 134mg
Sodium: 110mg
Total Carbs: 8.1g
Dietary Fiber: 2.3g
Protein: 15.3g

Paleo Spicy Shrimp Stir-Fry

"This flavorful stir-fry shrimp recipe is Paleo-friendly and flavored with ginger, lemon, and garlic."

Prep Time: 20 Minutes
Cook Time: 10 Minutes
Ready In: 8 Hours 30 Minutes
Servings: 4

INGREDIENTS:
1/2 cup lemon juice
1 small onion, finely chopped
1/2 cup olive oil
3 cloves garlic, minced
1 tablespoon lemon zest
1 tablespoon grated ginger
1 teaspoon ground turmeric
24 large shrimp, peeled and deveined
1 tablespoon coconut oil, or as needed

DIRECTIONS:
1. Mix together the turmeric, ginger, lemon zest, garlic, olive oil, onion, and lemon juice in a bowl.
2. Put the shrimp in the marinade you created in the step above, cover it, and refrigerate it overnight.
3. Remove the shrimp but save the marinade.
4. Heat a skillet or wok over medium-high heat and melt the coconut oil in it. Stir-fry the shrimp in the heated coconut oil for 5 to 10 minutes or until they are pink and opaque.
5. Add the reserved marinade and bring it to a boil and ensure that you stir the mixture constantly.

Ella Marie

NUTRITIONAL INFORMATION:
Servings Per Recipe: 4
Calories: 388
Amount Per Serving
Total Fat: 31.7g
Cholesterol: 192mg
Sodium: 222mg
Total Carbs: 5.9g
Dietary Fiber: 0.8g
Protein: 21.1g

Dinner

Paleo Chicken Stew

"This chicken stew is made with spinach and sweet potatoes, and you can adjust the amounts of chicken broth that you use to change its consistency."

Prep Time: 15 Minutes
Cook Time: 35 Minutes
Ready In: 50 Minutes
Servings: 6

INGREDIENTS:
2 teaspoons olive oil
2 garlic cloves, minced
1 small red onion, chopped
2 chicken breast halves, boneless, skinless, and cut into cubes
2 sweet potatoes, peeled, and chopped
1 cup fresh spinach, or to taste
1 pinch crushed red pepper, or more to taste
1 pinch paprika, or more to taste
Sea salt, to taste
1/2 cup chicken broth, or more to taste

DIRECTIONS:
1. Heat the olive oil over medium-high heat in a saucepan.
2. Sauté the garlic and onion for about 5 minutes in the heated olive oil until they soften.
3. Stir sea salt, paprika, crushed red pepper, spinach, sweet potatoes, and chicken with the onion and garlic in the saucepan.
4. Pour out as much chicken broth into the saucepan to make the mixture as stew-like or as soup-like as you desire.

5. Bring the broth to a boil, reduce the heat to medium-low and the mixture to simmer for half an hour or until the sweet potatoes are tender and the chicken is no longer pink in the middle.

NUTRITIONAL INFORMATION:
Servings Per Recipe: 6
Calories: 144
Amount Per Serving
Total Fat: 2.5g
Cholesterol: 21mg
Sodium: 207mg
Total Carbs: 20.8g
Dietary Fiber: 3.2g
Protein: 9.6g

Paleo Tilapia Dipped in Coconuts

"Tilapia fillets which have been dipped in coconuts are Paleo-friendly, tasty, and pan-fried in coconut oil. You can serve them with some tasty green vegetables!"

Prep Time: 15 Minutes
Cook Time: 10 Minutes
Ready In: 25 Minutes
Servings: 4

INGREDIENTS:
2 tablespoons coconut oil
Sea salt to taste
1/2 cup coconut flour
3/4 cup coconut, flaked and unsweetened
3 eggs, beaten
4 (4 ounce) tilapia fillets, or more as needed

DIRECTIONS:
1. Heat coconut oil over medium-high heat in a skillet.
2. Mix the salt, coconut flour, and unsweetened coconut together on a plate.
3. Brush the beaten egg over each tilapia fillet.
4. Press each fillet into coconut mixture so that it is evenly coated.
5. Gently toss the fillets between your hands so that the excess coconut pieces can fall off.
6. Place the coated fillets onto a plate and bread the rest but do not stack the fillets.
7. Fry the fillets in the hot oil for 5-7 minutes per side or until the fish flakes easily with a fork and until the fillets are golden brown.

Ella Marie

NUTRITIONAL INFORMATION:
Servings Per Recipe: 4
Calories: 462
Amount Per Serving
Total Fat: 26.5g
Cholesterol: 200mg
Sodium: 189mg
Total Carbs: 24.7g
Dietary Fiber: 15g
Protein: 32.9g

Spaghetti Carbonara-Paleo Style

"This Paleo-friendly Carbonara replaces pasta with spaghetti squash with tomatoes and bacon."

Prep Time: 10 Minutes
Cook Time: 50 Minutes
Ready In: 1 Hour
Servings: 4

INGREDIENTS:
1 spaghetti squash, large, halved, and seeded
1/4 cup extra-virgin olive oil
8 slices bacon, diced
1 teaspoon ground black pepper
1 teaspoon salt
1 large tomato, diced
4 large egg yolks
3 sprigs fresh basil

DIRECTIONS:
1. Preheat the oven to a temperature of 400°F (200°C).
2. Place the squash on a baking sheet cut side up.
3. Bake the squash in the preheated oven for 45-60 minutes until it becomes tender.
4. Scoop out the flesh of the squash and use a fork to shred it into strands.
5. Heat the olive oil over medium-high heat in a large skillet
6. Place the bacon in the hot oil and cook it and stir it for 5-10 minute or until it browned and thoroughly cooked through.
7. Add the shredded squash to the skillet and cook and stir it for 3-5 minutes or until the squash is softened.

8. Stir the pepper, salt, and the tomato into squash mixture and then remove the skillet from the heat.

9. Mix the egg yolks into the squash mixture until the mixture becomes creamy but do not allow the egg yolks to touch the skillet.

10. Transfer the squash Carbonara to a serving bowl and garnish it with the three fresh basil sprigs.

NUTRITIONAL INFORMATION:
Servings Per Recipe: 4
Calories: 428
Amount Per Serving
Total Fat: 28.7g
Cholesterol: 225mg
Sodium: 1091 mg
Total Carbs: 34.4g
Dietary Fiber: 0.7g
Protein: 12.9g

Paleo Broccoli Rabe and Sausage

"This Paleo-friendly recipe is a simple pan-frying of broccoli rabe and sausage which has been seasoned with lemon and garlic in some olive oil."

Prep Time: 10 Minutes
Cook Time: 20 Minutes
Ready In: 30 Minutes
Servings: 2

INGREDIENTS:
3 tablespoons divided olive oil, or more to taste
4 (3.5 ounce) links Italian sausage, sliced
2 large garlic cloves, minced
2 bunches broccoli rabe, trimmed
1 pinch lemon zest, or to taste
1 pinch ground red pepper, or to taste
Sea salt to taste
1/2 lemon

DIRECTIONS:
1. Coat the bottom of a skillet with a thin layer of olive oil.
2. Heat the skillet over medium heat.
3. Cook and stir the sausage slices for 3-5 minutes in skillet until they are browned
4. Add the garlic and continue cooking for an additional minute or until the garlic becomes fragrant.
5. Add the broccoli rabe to the skillet and season it with the sea salt, red pepper, and lemon zest.
6. Drizzle the olive oil over the broccoli rabe and toss it to coat it.

7. Cook the broccoli rabe whilst stirring occasionally for about 15 minutes or until it is completely wilted

8. Squeeze the lemon half all over the broccoli rabe and sausage mixture.

NUTRITIONAL INFORMATION:
Servings Per Recipe: 2
Calories: 688
Amount Per Serving
Total Fat: 54.6g
Cholesterol: 72 mg
Sodium: 1743 mg
Total Carbs: 18.7 g
Dietary Fiber: 6.4 g
Protein: 32.4g

OTHER WAYS OF TREATING LEPTIN RESISTANCE

Acupuncture

Acupuncture has been used in Traditional Chinese Medicine (TCM) for a very long time to treat a variety of disorders, but it has most recently proven useful in the treatment of Leptin resistance. It does this by aiding in weight loss.

Acupuncture helps to promote the release of endorphins, which are hormones in the body which make you feel calmer and more positive. It also helps to lessen the release of cortisol into the blood stream. This hormone disrupts digestion, contributes to depression, and may encourage emotional eating. When its concentration is reduced your body, you are less likely to put on weight and hence gain more fat cells which secrete even more Leptin into the blood.

In a study conducted by Turkish researchers on forty obese women, it was found that five weeks of acupuncture decreased the levels of Leptin and insulin in the blood, and this resulted in significant weight loss. Other studies conducted on other species yield the same results, so acupuncture can be a solution for many who are Leptin-resistant and overweight.

Intermittent Fasting

Intermittent fasting is a form of dietary restriction in which people alternate between periods of eating and periods of consuming nothing. It has been a part of some spiritual practices for ages, but recent studies have confirmed that there are numerous benefits that you can derive from fasting.

- Intermittent fasting lowers your triglyceride levels and, therefore, helps you to lose weight
- Intermittent fasting lessens the damage done by free radicals to your body and also reduces inflammation
- Intermittent fasting promotes human growth hormone (HGH) formation. Human growth hormone plays an important role in fitness, health, and slowing down the aging process.
- Intermittent fasting also helps to normalize Leptin levels in the body and, therefore, helps to improve Leptin sensitivity and reduce Leptin resistance
- Intermittent fasting helps to protect you from heart disease, diabetes, and even cancer because it helps to normalize blood insulin levels and improve your Leptin sensitivity.
- Intermittent fasting also increases catecholamines, which increase your resting energy expenditure while decreasing your insulin levels. This allows stored fat to be more easily burned as fuel.

Before you can understand how intermittent fasting helps you lose weight, I have to explain to you the difference between the fed state and the fasting state that your body goes through.

During the fed state, your body digests and absorbs food. This usually begins when you start eating and then lasts for three to five hours after the meal because your body continues to break down and absorb the food that you just ate. When you are in this state, it is very hard for you to lose weight by burning fat because your blood insulin levels are high.

After the three to five hours have elapsed, your body enters the post-absorptive state. This state lasts for eight to twelve hours after your last meal, and it is simply the state where your body is not processing a meal.

After this state, your body enters the fasting state. In this state is very easy for you to burn fat and lose weight because your blood insulin levels would be low and your body would easily use fat as an energy source. This is the reason why so many people who start to fast intermittently will lose body fat without changing their diets or their exercise habits.

Since we do not enter the fasting state until at least twelve hours after a meal, it is very rare that we will enter this state while we are on our normal eating plans without any direct efforts being made. Fasting helps to put our bodies in the state where it is optimized for burning fats as an energy source.

This reduction in fat will therefore reduce the quantity of Leptin being pumped into the blood, helping to increase Leptin sensitivity. After a while, you will find that fasting helps to normalize your Leptin levels and your blood glucose levels.

There are many different forms of intermittent fasting; you just have to choose the one that is right for you. Some of the more common forms include Leangains, Eat Stop Eat, The Warrior Diet, Fat Loss Forever, and The Alternate Day Fasting.

The Leangains diet demands that women fast for fourteen hours each day and men fast for sixteen hours. The rest of the time can be spent eating your normal food. You should not consume any calories during the fasting period however, but sugar-free gum, diet soda, calorie-free sweeteners, and black coffee are permitted. Most people fast through the night and then about six hours after they wake up. They then break the fast after this six-hour period has elapsed. Most people find this fasting program to be very flexible, but even though there is flexibility, the fasting program has very specific guidelines for what to eat. This strict nutrition plan may make this program harder to adhere to.

The Eat Stop Eat fasting plan demands that you fast for twenty four hours one or two times weekly. During the twenty-four-hour fasting period, you should not consume any calories, although calorie-free beverages are allowed. After you have completed your twenty-four hours, you many go back to your normal eating plan.

This fasting plan is also flexible, and there are no restrictions on what you can and cannot eat. Going twenty four hours without food can be very hard for some people, especially when they just start the dieting plan. This dieting plan may also cause fatigue, headaches, and anxiousness at first and it may also make some people cranky. The long fasting period may also make more people binge after the fast.

In the Warrior Diet fasting plan, you fast for about twenty hours daily and then eat a large meal at nighttime. There are guidelines on specifically what you should and should not eat during that large meal for the night, and there are also specific guidelines on the order in which you eat specific food groups. You should start with vegetables and then proteins and then fats. If you are still hungry after you finish those food groups, then you can consume some carbohydrates. During the twenty-hour fast, you are allowed to eat raw vegetables or fruits, a few servings of protein, or freshly squeezed juice. Many people like this fasting program because they are still allowed a few snacks during the fast, but there are specific guidelines to follow and strict schedules that can make it harder for some.

The Fat Loss Forever fasting plan takes the best part of the Leangains, Warrior Diet, and the Eat Stop Eat plan and combines them all to make one plan. With this fasting plan, you get one cheat day weekly, and that cheat day is followed by a thirty-six-hour fast. The rest of the seven-day cycle is split up between the different fasting plans. This plan is great for some because you get one whole cheat day, but this can pose a problem for many who may overeat on the cheat day. This plan may also be a bit confusing for some.

The Alternate Day fasting is pretty easy and self-explanatory: You eat very little one day and then eat normally the next day. More specifically, you eat one fifth of your normal calorie intake on the fasting day. This method has shown very impressive results where weight loss is concerned; some people have lost two and a half pounds per week by cutting their calories by 20%-35%. Many people may be tempted to binge on their normal eating day, however, so this can be disadvantage of this diet.

Other functions of Leptin in the body

Leptin is also an important hormone which helps to regulate the onset of puberty. It has been observed that undernourished and very thin females take longer to reach puberty than girls with more weight. In addition, very thin girls may not ovulate during their menstrual cycles, and some may never reach puberty, with their bodies remaining pre-pubescent for the rest of their lives.

Leptin also plays an important role in immunity, cardiovascular function, and bone metabolism. It has been shown that during an infection, Leptin levels rise drastically and then it decreases after the body returns to normal. It has been shown that persons with heart failure and certain other heart problems, such as cardiac cachexia, have low levels of Leptin circulating in their bloods. Leptin has been proven to promote bone formation in humans and other species. It stimulates the cells that make bones and aids in the formation of new blood vessels so that they can deliver nutrients to the newly-formed bone.

Conclusion

Leptin resistance is a serious complication that can escalate and lead to many other problems. It is caused by an excess of the Leptin hormone in the blood so that after a while the receptors for the Leptin hormone become unresponsive to its signal. There are many factors that can increase your resistance to Leptin, but that does not mean that it cannot be corrected. With the right behavioral and dietary changes, you can reverse your resistance to Leptin and many other hormones and get back your health, your fitness, and your life.

Did you Like "Leptin Resistance"?

Before you go, I'd like to say thank you so much for purchasing my book.

I know you could have picked from dozens of books on this subject, but you took a chance with mine, and I'm truly grateful for that. So, once again, a big thanks for downloading this book and reading all the way to the end—I truly appreciate it.

Now I'd like to ask for a small favor if you don't mind: Would you be so kind as to take a minute of your time and leave a review for this book on Amazon?

This feedback will help me continue to write the kind of books that help you get results. And if you loved it, then please feel free to let me know! :)

Printed in Great Britain
by Amazon.co.uk, Ltd.,
Marston Gate.

Leptin Resistance

The Ultimate Leptin Resistance Diet Guide For Weight Loss

Ella Marie

© 2015 Sender Publishing

© Copyright 2015 by Sender Publishing — All rights reserved.

This document is geared towards providing exact and reliable information in regards to the topic and issue covered. The publication is sold with the idea that the publisher is not required to render accounting, officially permitted, or otherwise, qualified services. If advice is necessary, legal or professional, a practiced individual in the profession should be ordered.

From a Declaration of Principles which was accepted and approved equally by a Committee of the American Bar Association and a Committee of Publishers and Associations.

In no way is it legal to reproduce, duplicate, or transmit any part of this document in either electronic means or in printed format. Recording of this publication is strictly prohibited and any storage of this document is not allowed unless with written permission from the publisher. All rights reserved.

The information provided herein is stated to be truthful and consistent, in that any liability, in terms of inattention or otherwise, by any usage or abuse of any policies, processes, or directions contained within is the solitary and utter responsibility of the recipient reader. Under no circumstances will any legal responsibility or blame be held against the publisher for any reparation, damages, or monetary loss due to the information herein, either directly or indirectly.

Respective authors own all copyrights not held by the publisher.

The information herein is offered for informational purposes solely, and is universal as so. The presentation of the information is without contract or any type of guarantee assurance.

The ideas, concepts and/or opinions delivered in this book are to be used for educational purposes only. This book is provided with the understanding that authors and publisher are not rendering medical advice of any kind, nor is this book intended to replace medical advice, nor to diagnose, prescribe or treat any disease, condition, illness or injury.

It is imperative that before beginning any diet or exercise program, including any aspect of this book, you receive full medical clearance from a licensed doctor and/or physician. Author and publisher claim no responsibility to any person or entity for any liability, loss, or damage caused or alleged to be caused directly or indirectly as a result of the use, application or interpretation of the material in this book.

The trademarks that are used are without any consent, and the publication of the trademark is without permission or backing by the trademark owner. All trademarks and brands within this book are for clarifying purposes only and are owned by the owners themselves, not affiliated with this document.

Table of Contents

Introduction 1
First things First: What is Leptin? 2
What is Leptin Resistance and How It Works 6
Causes of Leptin Resistance 9
Signs of Leptin Resistance 13
Treating Leptin Resistance Naturally 14
Meal Ideas 23
Other Ways of Treating Leptin Resistance 47
Other Functions of Leptin in the Body 52
Conclusion 53